Journey to a Healthier Me: A Weight loss Story

ANDRE RODGERS

Contents

Journey to a Healthier Me: A Weight Loss Story

Sometimes, the most profound conversations we have are the ones with ourselves. It was during one of these introspective moments that I realized I needed to make a change. I took a hard look at my lifestyle, health habits, and overall well-being.

In that quiet moment, I asked myself some tough questions. Was I truly happy with my current state? Was I doing everything I could to take care of myself? The answers were a wake-up call. I acknowledged that I wasn't just dissatisfied with my weight, but also with the lack of energy and confidence it brought.

This conversation with myself was a turning point. It made me realize that I had the power to change my narrative. I understood that the journey to a healthier me was not just about losing weight; it was about reclaiming my life, my vitality, and my happiness. With a newfound determination, I decided to embark on a weight-loss journey.

I set realistic goals, researched healthier eating habits, and found exercise routines that I enjoyed. I reminded myself that this journey would be challenging but worthwhile. Each small step forward was a victory, and each setback was a lesson.

The internal dialogue that sparked this journey was a reminder of my strength and resilience. It motivated me to prioritize my health and well-being, and to never underestimate the power of self-reflection and self-motivation.

Introduction

Embarking on a weight-loss journey is a deeply personal and transformative experience. This book is designed to guide, inspire, and support you through the highs and lows of shedding pounds and gaining a healthier, more fulfilling life.

Andre Rodgers

Chapter 1

Understanding Your Why

Finding Your Motivation

Understanding your "why" and finding motivation for weight loss are crucial steps in achieving and maintaining your health goals. Here's how you can explore and solidify your motivation:

Identifying Your "Why"

1. Reflect on Personal Reasons:

>   Health: Consider health-related reasons such as reducing the risk of chronic diseases (diabetes, heart disease, etc.), improving mobility, or managing existing conditions.

>   Energy and Vitality: Think about how weight loss can enhance your daily energy levels and overall vitality.

>   Longevity: Reflect on the desire to live a longer, healthier life for yourself and your loved ones.

2. Emotional and Psychological Factors:

> Self-Esteem: Consider how weight loss might improve your self-esteem and confidence.

> Mental Health: Reflect on the potential positive impact on mental health, including reduced anxiety or depression.

> Stress Relief: Recognize how adopting a healthier lifestyle can help in managing stress.

3. Social and Lifestyle Motivations:

> Family and Friends: Think about being more active and present for family activities or setting a positive example for loved ones.

> Social Life: Consider how weight loss can improve your social interactions and experiences.

> Personal Goals: Reflect on specific personal goals like fitting into certain clothes, preparing for an event (wedding, reunion), or achieving a fitness milestone.

Finding and Sustaining Motivation

1. Set Clear, Achievable Goals:

> Short-Term Goals: Establish small, realistic goals that are attainable in the short term, providing regular milestones to celebrate.

> Long-Term Goals: Define long-term objectives that align with your "why" and provide a vision for your future health and well-being.

2. Create a Support System:

Accountability Partners: Find friends, family members, or a support group who can encourage you and hold you accountable.

Professional Support: Consider seeking help from health professionals like dietitians, personal trainers, or therapists. It is also important to discuss your plans with your primary care physician (PCP), especially if you have any medical conditions such as diabetes or hypertension. Finding a functional medicine PCP can be particularly beneficial, as they focus on nutritional health and understand the interactions of various forms of nutrition and supplements. Functional medicine PCPs receive extensive training in nutrition and its potential for healing and prevention, beyond just treating symptoms with medications. Personally, my health significantly improved once I found a functional medicine PCP.

3. Track Progress and Celebrate Milestones:

Monitoring: Use tools like journals, apps, or trackers to monitor your progress. It's also important to express heartfelt gratitude and appreciation for each achievement, no matter how small. Gratitude journaling can be a powerful tool in this process, helping to maintain a positive mindset and reinforcing your commitment to your goals.

Celebrate Successes: Recognize and celebrate each milestone, no matter how small, to maintain motivation.

4. Develop a Positive Mindset:

> Self-Compassion: Practice self-compassion and understand that setbacks are a part of the journey.

> Positive Reinforcement: Use positive reinforcement to keep your morale high and stay focused on your achievements. Incorporating a gratitude practice can also be beneficial, as regularly expressing gratitude for your progress and efforts helps reinforce a positive mindset and sustain motivation.

5. Integrate Enjoyable Activities:

> Exercise You Love: Choose physical activities that you enjoy, making it easier to stay consistent.

> Tasty, Healthy Foods: Explore and incorporate healthy foods that you find delicious and satisfying.

By deeply understanding your "why" and actively finding ways to maintain motivation, you can create a strong foundation for a successful and sustainable weight-loss journey.

The importance of a strong, personal reason for losing weight.

Having a strong personal reason for losing weight is crucial for several reasons:

1. Provides Direction and Purpose

> Clarity: A clear personal reason gives you a sense of purpose and direction. It helps you understand why you are making changes to your lifestyle.

Focus: Knowing your "why" helps you stay focused on your goals, especially when faced with challenges or temptations.

2. Enhances Motivation and Commitment

Intrinsic Motivation: Personal reasons are often deeply rooted and provide intrinsic motivation, which is more sustainable than external motivators like societal pressure or superficial desires.

Resilience: A strong personal reason can help you stay committed during tough times, increasing your resilience against setbacks.

3. Increases Likelihood of Long-Term Success

Sustainable Habits: When your motivation is deeply personal, you are more likely to develop habits that are sustainable in the long term, rather than relying on quick fixes.

Consistency: Personal reasons help you maintain consistency in your efforts, which is key to achieving and maintaining weight loss.

4. Improves Emotional and Psychological Well-Being

Self-Esteem: Pursuing weight loss for personal reasons often aligns with improving self-esteem and body image.

Mental Health: Achieving goals tied to personal values can enhance mental health and overall well-being.

5. Strengthens Resolve and Decision-Making

Better Choices: With a strong personal reason, you are more likely to make healthier choices that align with your goals.

Prioritization: It helps you prioritize your health and well-being, making it easier to avoid distractions and stay on track.

6. Personal Empowerment

Sense of Control: Understanding and embracing your personal reasons for weight loss empowers you to take control of your health journey.

Confidence: Achieving goals that are personally meaningful boosts your confidence and reinforces your ability to make positive changes.

7. Alignment with Personal Values and Beliefs

Consistency: When your weight-loss goals align with your core values and beliefs, your actions are more consistent with who you are, leading to greater fulfillment.

Authenticity: Pursuing weight loss for reasons that resonate with your true self fosters a sense of authenticity and genuine satisfaction.

Practical Steps to Identify and Strengthen Your Personal Reason

1. Reflect on Your Motivations: Spend time thinking about why you want to lose weight and how it aligns with your overall life goals.

2. Write It Down: Document your reasons and keep them visible to remind yourself regularly.

3. Visualize Success: Imagine how achieving your weight-loss goals will positively impact your life.

4. Set Specific Goals: Break down your personal reasons into specific, measurable goals.

5. Seek Support: Share your reasons with trusted friends or family members who can provide encouragement and accountability.

In summary, a strong personal reason for losing weight is vital as it fuels motivation, enhances commitment, and supports long-term success by aligning your actions with your intrinsic values and goals.

Journaling your Thoughts and Goals

Journaling can be a powerful tool for weight loss, helping you to clarify your thoughts, set goals, track progress, and stay motivated. Here are some tips and prompts to help you get started with weight-loss journaling:

Benefits of Journaling for Weight Loss

1. Clarity and Focus:

Organizing Thoughts: Writing down your thoughts helps you organize and make sense of them.

Setting Clear Goals: Journaling allows you to articulate and refine your weight-loss goals.

2. Accountability:

Tracking Progress: Regularly recording your progress helps you stay accountable to your goals.

Identifying Patterns: Journaling can help you identify patterns in your eating and exercise habits, as well as emotional triggers.

3. Emotional Processing:

Managing Emotions: Writing about your feelings can help you process emotions that might be affecting your weight-loss journey.

Building Resilience: Reflecting on challenges and successes helps build resilience and a positive mindset.

4. Motivation and Inspiration:

Celebrating Successes: Recording achievements, no matter how small, keeps you motivated.

Reflecting on Your "Why": Revisiting your reasons for losing weight can reinforce your commitment.

How to Start Journaling for Weight Loss

1. Choose a Journal:

Digital or Paper: Decide whether you prefer a digital journal (apps, documents) or a physical notebook.

Format: Consider structured formats (prompt-based) or freeform styles, depending on what suits you best.

2. Set a Routine:

Consistency: Aim to journal regularly, whether daily, weekly, or at specific times (e.g., after meals or workouts).

Time of Day: Choose a time that works best for you, such as in the morning to set intentions or in the evening to reflect on the day, or both.

Journal Prompts for Weight Loss

1. Setting Goals:

Short-Term Goals: What are my weight-loss goals for the next week/month?

Long-Term Goals: What do I hope to achieve in the next six months/year?

2. Reflecting on Motivation:

Personal Reasons: Why do I want to lose weight? What are my most compelling reasons?

Future Benefits: How will my life improve as I reach my weight-loss goals?

3. Daily Entries:

Meals and Snacks: What did I eat today? How did I feel before, during, and after eating?

Physical Activity: What exercise did I do today? How did it make me feel?

Emotions and Triggers: What emotions did I experience today? Did any triggers affect my eating habits?

4. Progress and Milestones:

Achievements: What successes have I achieved recently? What small victories can I celebrate?

Challenges: What obstacles have I faced? How did I handle them? What can I learn from them?

5. Self-Reflection:

Body Image: How do I feel about my body today? How is my body changing?

Mindset: What positive thoughts can I focus on today? How can I stay motivated?

6. Planning Ahead:

Meal Planning: What healthy meals can I prepare this week?

Exercise Planning: What physical activities can I schedule for the week ahead?

Tips for Effective Journaling

1. Be Honest and Compassionate:

Honesty: Be truthful with yourself in your journal entries. Acknowledge both strengths and areas for improvement.

Compassion: Treat yourself with kindness. Use your journal as a space for self-compassion, not self-criticism.

2. Include Details:

Specifics: Include specific details about your meals, activities, and emotions. This will help you identify patterns and make necessary adjustments.

3. Reflect and Adjust:

Regular Review: Regularly review your journal entries to reflect on your progress and make adjustments to your plan as needed.

Adaptability: Be flexible and willing to change your goals and strategies based on your reflections and insights.

4. Use Positive Reinforcement:

Celebrate: Celebrate your successes and milestones. Acknowledge your efforts and progress, no matter how small.

Example Journal Entry

Date: June 24, 2024

Goals for Today:
Eat balanced meals with plenty of vegetables and protein.
Walk for at least 30 minutes.
Practice mindful eating during meals.

Meals:
Breakfast: Oatmeal with berries and nuts. Felt satisfied and energized.
Lunch: Grilled chicken salad with a variety of veggies. Felt good about making a healthy choice.
Dinner: Stir-fried tofu with broccoli and brown rice. Enjoyed the flavors and felt full.
Snacks: Apple slices and a handful of almonds. Helped curb my hunger between meals.

Exercise:
Walked for 45 minutes in the park. Enjoyed the fresh air and felt more relaxed afterward.

Emotions and Reflections:
Felt a bit stressed about work today, but the walk helped clear my mind. Proud of my food choices today; I stuck to my plan and felt in control.

Successes and Challenges:
Success: Met my exercise goal and ate balanced meals.
Challenge: Felt a craving for sweets after dinner but opted for a healthy snack instead.

Plan for Tomorrow:
Prepare a healthy lunch to take to work.
Do a 20-minute yoga session in the morning.

By incorporating these strategies and prompts into your journaling practice, you can create a powerful tool to support your weight-loss journey, providing clarity, motivation, and a deeper understanding of your personal progress.

Setting Realistic Goals: Long-term vs. short-term goals.

Setting realistic long-term and short-term goals for weight loss is essential for maintaining motivation, tracking progress, and achieving sustainable results.

Here's how to effectively set and balance these goals:

Short-Term Goals

Short-term goals are achievable within a few weeks to a couple of months. They help create momentum and provide immediate rewards, keeping you motivated.

Examples of Short-Term Goals:

1. Weekly Weight-Loss Targets:
Aim to lose 1-2 pounds per week, a healthy and sustainable rate.

2. Dietary Changes:
Incorporate five servings of fruits and vegetables daily.
Reduce intake of sugary beverages and replace them with water or herbal teas.

3. Exercise Goals:
Exercise for at least 30 minutes, five days a week.
Try a new workout class or physical activity each month.

4. Behavioral Goals:
Practice mindful eating during each meal.
Keep a daily food and exercise journal.

5. Hydration:
Drink at least 8 glasses of water daily.

How to Set Short-Term Goals:

1. Specific: Clearly define what you want to achieve (e.g., walk 10,000 steps daily).

2. Measurable: Ensure your goal can be tracked (e.g., lose 5 pounds in a month).

3. Achievable: Set a goal that is realistic given your current lifestyle and commitments.

4. Relevant: Choose goals that align with your long-term objectives.

5. Time-Bound: Set a deadline for achieving your goal (e.g., by the end of the month).

Long-Term Goals

Long-term goals are broader and take several months to a year or more to achieve. They provide a vision for where you want to be and help maintain focus over an extended period.

Examples of Long-Term Goals:

1. Weight Loss:
   - Lose 50 pounds in one year.
2. Health Improvements:
   - Lower blood pressure or cholesterol levels within six months.
   - Improve overall fitness to run a 5K race in nine months.
3. Lifestyle Changes:
   - Develop a sustainable, balanced diet that you enjoy and can maintain indefinitely.
   - Establish a regular exercise routine that includes a variety of activities.

4. Body Composition:
   - Reduce body fat percentage by a specific amount over the next year.

Setting realistic long-term and short-term goals for weight loss is essential for maintaining motivation, tracking progress, and achieving sustainable results.

How to Set Long-Term Goals:

1. Vision-Oriented: Focus on your ultimate aspirations (e.g., achieving a healthy BMI).

2. Broad and Comprehensive: Encompass various aspects of your health and lifestyle (e.g., diet, exercise, mental health).

3. Flexible: Be prepared to adjust your goals as you progress and circumstances change.

4.   Inspiring: Choose goals that are meaningful and motivate you to persist through challenges.

5.   Commitment: Recognize that long-term goals require sustained effort and dedication.

Balancing Short-Term and Long-Term Goals

1. Align Short-Term Goals with Long-Term Vision:
   - Ensure that your short-term goals are steppingstones that lead to your long-term objectives. For example, if your long-term goal is to lose 50 pounds in a year, short-term goals might include losing 4-5 pounds per month.

2. Regular Assessment and Adjustment:
   - Periodically review your goals and progress. Adjust your short-term goals based on your achievements and any changes in your circumstances.

3. Celebrate Milestones:
   - Recognize and celebrate when you achieve short-term goals. This boosts motivation and helps maintain focus on your long-term objectives.

4. Stay Flexible and Adapt:
   - Life can be unpredictable. Be prepared to adapt both short-term and long-term goals as needed to stay on track.

5. Use Short-Term Successes to Build Momentum:
   - Use the achievement of short-term goals to build confidence and momentum toward reaching your long-term goals.

Example of Integrated Goal Setting

Long-Term Goal: Lose 50 pounds in one year.

Short-Term Goals:

- Month 1: Lose 5 pounds by eating balanced meals and walking 30 minutes daily.
- Month 2: Continue losing 4-5 pounds by incorporating strength training twice a week.
- Month 3: Reduce intake of processed foods and increase water intake to 10 glasses daily.
- Month 6: Participate in a local 5K walk/run event.
- Month 9: Join a fitness class to add variety to your routine.

By effectively setting and balancing realistic short-term and long-term goals, you create a structured path to follow, which helps maintain motivation, track progress, and achieve sustainable weight loss results.

How to Set Long-Term Goals:

1. Vision-Oriented: Focus on your ultimate aspirations (e.g., achieving a healthy BMI).

2. Broad and Comprehensive: Encompass various aspects of your health and lifestyle (e.g., diet, exercise, mental health).

3. Flexible: Be prepared to adjust your goals as you progress and circumstances change.

4. Inspiring: Choose goals that are meaningful and motivate you to persist through challenges.

5. Commitment: Recognize that long-term goals require sustained effort and dedication.

The significance of measurable and achievable targets.

Chapter 2

The Basics of Nutrition

Understanding Calories and Macros

Calories: The Basics

Think of calories as the fuel your body needs to keep moving. Just like a car needs gas, you need calories for energy. Too much fuel, and your car's tank overflows. Too few, and you're running on empty. Finding the right balance is key to keeping your engine (body) running smoothly.

Macronutrients: Proteins, Carbohydrates, and Fats

Macronutrients, or "macros," are the building blocks of your diet. Let's break them down:

1. Proteins: Imagine proteins as the construction workers of your body. They build and repair tissues, helping you stay strong. Foods like chicken, beans, and tofu are packed with these mighty builders.

2. Carbohydrates: Think of carbs as your body's favorite fuel. They power your brain and muscles, especially during work-outs. Whole grains, fruits, and veggies are great sources of these energy boosters.

3. Fats: Fats are like the lubricants that keep your engine running smoothly. They support cell function and help you absorb vitamins. Avocados, nuts, and olive oil are some tasty options to keep things running efficiently.

By understanding the basics of calories and macros, you're setting the stage for a healthier, more energized you! Ready to dive deeper into building a balanced diet and making meal planning fun? Let's go!

Chapter 3

The Role of Exercise

Finding an Activity You Enjoy

Exploring different types of exercise.

The benefits of both cardio and strength training.

The Role of Exercise in a Weight-loss Journey

Exercise is a critical component of a successful weight-loss journey. It not only helps you burn calories but also improves your overall health, boosts your mood, and increases your energy levels. Here's how to incorporate exercise effectively into your routine:

Finding an Activity You Enjoy

1. Experiment with Different Activities: Try various forms of exercise to discover what you enjoy the most. This could include running, swimming, cycling, dancing, hiking, or group fitness classes.

2. Combine Fun and Fitness: Activities like playing a sport, joining a dance class, or hiking with friends can make exercise feel less like a chore and more like a fun hobby.

3.   Stay Open-Minded: Be willing to try new things. Sometimes, an activity you never considered might become your favorite way to stay active.

Exploring Different Types of Exercise

1. Cardiovascular (Cardio) Exercise:

Examples: Running, cycling, swimming, brisk walking, aerobics, and jump rope.

Benefits: Improves heart and lung health, boosts metabolism, and burns a significant number of calories.

2. Strength Training:

Examples: Weightlifting, resistance band exercises, bodyweight exercises (like push-ups and squats), and Pilates.

Benefits: Builds muscle mass, increases metabolic rate, strengthens bones, and enhances overall body strength and posture.

3. Flexibility and Balance Training:

Examples: Yoga, Pilates, and stretching routines.

Benefits: Improves flexibility, reduces the risk of injury, enhances balance and coordination, and can aid in muscle recovery.

Benefits of Both Cardio and Strength Training

Cardiovascular Exercise

1. Calorie Burning: Cardio exercises are effective for burning calories, which helps create the calorie deficit needed for weight loss.

2. Heart Health: Regular cardio strengthens the heart and improves cardiovascular health, reducing the risk of heart disease.

3. Endurance and Stamina: Cardio boosts your endurance and stamina, making daily activities easier and less tiring.

4. Mental Health: Cardio exercise releases endorphins, which can improve mood and reduce symptoms of anxiety and depression.

Strength Training

1. Increased Metabolism: Building muscle through strength training increases your resting metabolic rate, meaning you burn more calories even at rest.

2. Body Composition: Strength training helps you build lean muscle mass, which can improve your body composition and give you a more toned appearance.

3. Bone Health: Weight-bearing exercises strengthen bones and can help prevent osteoporosis.

4. Functional Strength: Enhances your ability to perform every-day tasks, reducing the risk of injuries and improving quality of life.

Creating a Balanced Exercise Routine

1. Mix Cardio and Strength: Aim to include both cardio and strength training in your weekly routine. For example, you might do cardio three days a week and strength training two days a week.

2. Include Rest Days: Allow for adequate recovery by incorporating rest days or light activity days to prevent overtraining and injury.

3. Progress Gradually: Gradually increase the intensity, duration, or frequency of your workouts to continue challenging your body and making progress.

Sample Weekly Exercise Plan

Monday
Cardio: 30-minute run or brisk walk

Tuesday
Strength Training: Full-body workout (e.g., squats, lunges, push-ups, rows, and planks)

Wednesday
Cardio: 30-minute cycling or swimming

Thursday
Strength Training: Upper body focus (e.g., dumbbell presses, bicep curls, tricep dips, shoulder presses)

Friday
Cardio: 30-minute dance class or aerobics

Saturday
Strength Training: Lower body focus (e.g., deadlifts, leg presses, calf raises, glute bridges)

Sunday
Flexibility and Balance: Yoga or stretching routine

Staying Motivated

1. Set Realistic Goals: Define clear and achievable fitness goals to keep yourself motivated.

2. Track Progress: Keep a workout journal or use fitness apps to track your progress and celebrate milestones.

3. Find a Workout Buddy: Exercising with a friend can provide accountability, support, and make workouts more enjoyable.

4. Variety and Fun: Regularly change your routine to keep things interesting and prevent boredom.

By finding exercises you enjoy and incorporating both cardio and strength training into your routine, you can enhance your weight-loss efforts and improve your overall health and well-being.

Creating a Workout Routine
Starting slow and building up.

Incorporating variety to stay motivated.
Creating a Workout Routine for Weight Loss

Starting slow and gradually building up your workout routine is a smart strategy, especially if you're new to exercising or returning after a break. This approach helps prevent injury, allows your body to adapt, and makes the process more enjoyable. Incorporating variety keeps you motivated and engaged.

Week 1-2: Starting Slow

Goal: Build a foundation and establish a habit of regular exercise.

Frequency: 3-4 days per week

Workouts:

1. Cardio:
   Activity: Brisk walking
   Duration: 20-30 minutes
   Frequency: 2 times per week

2. Strength Training:
   Activity: Bodyweight exercises
   Duration: 20 minutes
   Frequency: 2 times per week
   Exercises:
        Squats: 2 sets of 10-12 reps
        Push-ups (on knees if needed): 2 sets of 8-10 reps
        Plank: 2 sets of 20-30 seconds
        Glute bridges: 2 sets of 10-12 reps

3. Flexibility and Balance:
   Activity: Stretching or yoga
   Duration: 10-15 minutes
   Frequency: 1-2 times per week

Week 3-4: Building Up

Goal: Increase intensity and duration, introduce more variety.

Frequency: 4-5 days per week

Workouts:

1. Cardio:
   Activity: Walking, jogging, or cycling
   Duration: 30-40 minutes
   Frequency: 2-3 times per week
   Variation: Alternate between brisk walking and light jogging (intervals)

2. Strength Training:
   Activity: Bodyweight and light weights/resistance bands
   Duration: 30 minutes
   Frequency: 2 times per week
   Exercises:
      Squats: 3 sets of 12-15 reps
      Push-ups: 3 sets of 10-12 reps
      Plank: 3 sets of 30-45 seconds
      Glute bridges: 3 sets of 12-15 reps
      Resistance band rows: 3 sets of 12-15 reps

3. Flexibility and Balance:
   Activity: Yoga or dynamic stretching
   Duration: 15-20 minutes
   Frequency: 1-2 times per week

Week 5-8: Increasing Variety and Intensity

Goal: Add more variety and challenge to your routine.

Frequency: 5-6 days per week

Workouts:

1. Cardio:
   Activity: Running, swimming, cycling, or group fitness classes (e.g., Zumba, kickboxing)
   Duration: 40-45 minutes
   Frequency: 3 times per week
   Variation: Include interval training (e.g., 1-minute sprint, 2-minute walk, repeat)

2. Strength Training:
   Activity: Free weights, machines, or advanced bodyweight exercises
   Duration: 35-45 minutes
   Frequency: 3 times per week
   Exercises:
       Squats: 3 sets of 15-20 reps (add weight if comfortable)
       Push-ups: 3 sets of 15-20 reps
       Plank: 3 sets of 45-60 seconds
       Glute bridges: 3 sets of 15-20 reps
       Dumbbell rows: 3 sets of 12-15 reps
       Lunges: 3 sets of 12-15 reps per leg

3. Flexibility and Balance:
   Activity: Yoga, Pilates, or Tai Chi
   Duration: 20-30 minutes
   Frequency: 2 times per week

Tips for Incorporating Variety

1. Mix Up Cardio: Alternate between different types of cardio exercises like running, cycling, swimming, and dance classes to keep things fresh.

2. Try New Classes: Participate in group fitness classes like kick-boxing, spinning, or HIIT to add variety and meet new people.

3. Use Different Equipment: Incorporate dumbbells, resistance bands, kettlebells, and stability balls into your strength training.

4. Change Locations: Work out in different environments, such as parks, gyms, home, or community centers, to keep your routine exciting.

5. Interval Training: Combine high-intensity intervals with lower-intensity recovery periods to boost calorie burn and add variety.

6. Workout Challenges: Set short-term challenges, like a 30-day squat challenge or a plank challenge, to keep yourself motivated and focused.

Sample Weekly Workout Plan

Monday
Cardio: 30-minute run/walk intervals
Flexibility: 15-minute stretching routine

Tuesday
Strength Training: Full-body workout (35 minutes)

Wednesday
Cardio: 40-minute cycling
Flexibility: 15-minute yoga

Thursday
Strength Training: Upper body workout (35 minutes)

Friday
Cardio: 45-minute dance class or aerobics

Saturday
Strength Training: Lower body workout (40 minutes)
Flexibility: 20-minute Pilates

Sunday
Active Rest: Light activity like walking, playing a sport, or gentle yoga

By starting slow, gradually building up, and incorporating a variety of exercises, you can create a sustainable and enjoyable workout routine that supports your weight-loss journey and keeps you motivated.

Chapter 4

The Mental Game

Building a Positive Mindset

Overcoming self-doubt and negative thinking.

The mental aspect of a weight-loss journey is often as important as the physical changes. Building a positive mindset and overcoming self-doubt and negative thinking can significantly influence your success. Here are strategies to help you develop a strong mental game:

Building A Positive Mindset

1. Set Realistic and Achievable Goals

> SMART Goals: Use the SMART criteria (Specific, Measurable, Achievable, Relevant, Time-bound) to set clear and attainable goals. This approach makes it easier to track progress and stay motivated.

> Short-Term and Long-Term Goals: Break your long-term weight-loss goal into smaller, manageable short-term goals. Celebrate these small victories to keep your motivation high.

2. Visualize Success

Positive Visualization: Spend a few minutes each day visualizing yourself achieving your weight-loss goals. Imagine how you will look and feel, and the benefits you will enjoy.

Vision Board: Create a vision board with images and quotes that represent your goals and motivations. Place it where you can see it daily as a reminder of your objectives.

3. Practice Gratitude

On your journey to a healthier you, practicing gratitude should include quietly saying thank you for each thing you encounter during the day that you appreciate, as well as thanking other people when appropriate. For gratitude to be truly effective, it needs to be part of your entire mindset. Adopting "an attitude of gratitude" as a way of life can significantly enhance your overall well-being.

Gratitude Journal: Keep a gratitude journal where you write down things you are thankful for each day. Focusing on the positive aspects of your life can improve your overall mindset and keep you motivated.

Positive Affirmations: Use positive affirmations to boost your self-esteem and confidence. Repeat affirmations like, "I am capable of achieving my goals," or "I am becoming healthier every day."

4. Celebrate Progress

Non-Scale Victories: Celebrate non-scale victories such as increased energy levels, improved fitness, better sleep, and healthier habits. These milestones are important indicators of progress.

Reward Yourself: Reward yourself with non-food treats, such as a new workout outfit, a spa day, or a fun activity, when you reach a goal.

Overcoming Self-Doubt and Negative Thinking

1. Identify Negative Thoughts

Awareness: Pay attention to your inner dialogue and identify negative thoughts or self-doubt. Awareness is the first step to overcoming these thoughts.

Challenge Negative Thoughts: Question the validity of negative thoughts. Are they based on facts or assumptions? Replace them with more balanced and positive thoughts.

2. Reframe Your Mindset

Growth Mindset: Adopt a growth mindset, which emphasizes that abilities and intelligence can be developed with effort and learning. View challenges and setbacks as opportunities to grow and improve.

Positive Self-Talk: Replace negative self-talk with positive self-talk. Instead of saying, "I can't do this," say, "I am learning and getting better every day."

3. Focus on What You Can Control

Control the Controllable: Focus on the aspects of your weight-loss journey that you can control, such as your eating habits, exercise routine, and mindset. Let go of things outside your control, like genetic factors or temporary setbacks.

Take Action: Take proactive steps towards your goals, no matter how small. Action builds momentum and can help dispel self-doubt.

4. Seek Support

Social Support: Surround yourself with supportive friends, family, or join a weight-loss support group. Sharing your journey with others can provide encouragement and accountability.

Professional Help: Consider seeking help from a therapist or counselor if negative thinking and self-doubt are significantly impacting your progress.

5. Learn from Setbacks

Reflect and Adjust: View setbacks as learning opportunities rather than failures. Reflect on what went wrong, adjust your approach, and keep moving forward.

Resilience: Build resilience by developing coping strategies for dealing with setbacks and stress. Techniques like mindfulness, meditation, and deep breathing can help manage stress and keep you focused.

Example Strategies to Apply

1. Daily Affirmations and Visualization

Every morning, spend 5 minutes practicing positive affirmations and visualizing your success. Picture yourself reaching your weight-loss goals and experiencing the benefits.

2. Gratitude Journal

At the end of each day, write down three things you are grateful for. This practice helps shift your focus from what's going wrong to what's going right.

3. Reframe Negative Thoughts

When you catch yourself thinking negatively, stop and reframe the thought. For example, if you think, "I'll never lose this weight," reframe it to, "I am making progress every day and will reach my goals with patience and effort."

4. Set Achievable Mini-Goals

Instead of focusing solely on a large goal, set mini-goals such as losing 5 pounds, drinking more water daily, or walking for 30 minutes three times a week. Achieving these smaller goals will build confidence and momentum.

5. Support System

Share your goals and progress with a friend or family member who can provide encouragement and hold you accountable. Join an online community or local support group for additional motivation.

By incorporating these strategies into your daily routine, you can build a positive mindset, overcome self-doubt, and maintain motivation throughout your weight-loss journey. Remember, mental strength is a crucial component of achieving long-term success in any endeavor.

Practicing Mindfulness and Self-Compassion

Coping with Setbacks and Viewing Setbacks as Learning Opportunities.

Coping with setbacks in your weight-loss journey is crucial for maintaining long-term success and developing a healthy mindset. Viewing setbacks as learning opportunities can help you stay motivated and resilient. Here's how to effectively cope with setbacks and turn them into valuable lessons:

Coping with Setbacks

1. Acknowledge the Setback:

> Recognize and accept that setbacks are a natural part of any weight-loss journey. It's important to acknowledge them without judgment.

2. Reflect on the Cause:

> Take time to reflect on what caused the setback. Was it stress, lack of planning, emotional eating, or something else? Identifying the cause can help you understand what needs to be addressed.

3. Practice Self-Compassion:

> Be kind to yourself. Everyone makes mistakes, and it's important to treat yourself with the same kindness and understanding you would offer a friend.

4. Reassess Your Goals:

Revisit your weight-loss goals and ensure they are realistic and attainable. Adjust them if necessary to better fit your current situation.

5. Create a Plan:

Develop a specific plan to get back on track. This might include setting new short-term goals, planning meals, scheduling exercise, or seeking support from friends or a professional.

Viewing Setbacks as Learning Opportunities

1. Identify Lessons Learned:

Each setback provides an opportunity to learn something new about yourself and your habits. Ask yourself what you can learn from the experience and how you can use this knowledge to avoid similar setbacks in the future.

2. Focus on Progress, Not Perfection:

Remember that progress is more important than perfection. Celebrate your successes, no matter how small, and view setbacks as temporary detours rather than failures.

3. Develop Problem-Solving Skills:

Use setbacks to enhance your problem-solving skills. For example, if you tend to overeat when stressed, explore stress management techniques such as meditation, exercise, or talking to a friend.

4. Stay Positive and Motivated:

Keep a positive attitude and remind yourself why you started your weight-loss journey. Visualize your goals and focus on the benefits of achieving them.

Practical Tips for Moving Forward

1. Journal Your Experience:

Write about your setbacks in a journal. Include what happened, how you felt, and what you learned. This can help you process your emotions and gain insights.

2. Seek Support:

Don't hesitate to reach out for support. Talk to friends, family, or join a support group. Sometimes, sharing your experiences with others can provide comfort and encouragement.

3. Implement Small Changes:

Start with small, manageable changes to regain momentum. For example, if you missed several workouts, begin with short, easy exercises to build back your routine.

4. Focus on Healthy Habits:

Concentrate on building healthy habits rather than solely on the number on the scale. Consistent healthy eating, regular physical activity, and sufficient sleep are key components of weight loss and overall well-being.

5. Visualize Success:

Visualization can be a powerful tool. Spend a few minutes each day visualizing yourself achieving your goals and experiencing the benefits of your weight-loss journey.

Example of Turning a Setback into a Learning Opportunity

Situation: You went on vacation and indulged in unhealthy foods, resulting in weight gain.

Reflection:

Identify the Cause: Lack of healthy food options, being in a vacation mindset, and not exercising.

Lesson Learned: Planning ahead can help manage food choices, and incorporating physical activity during vacations is important.

Plan for the Future:

Pre-Trip Planning: Research healthy food options at your destination and plan to bring along some healthy snacks.

Mindful Eating: Practice mindful eating even while enjoying treats.

Stay Active: Incorporate physical activities like walking, swimming, or hiking into your vacation plans.

Positive Outcome:

> You now have a better strategy for managing your diet and exercise during future vacations.

> By viewing setbacks as learning opportunities, you can develop a more resilient and positive mindset, which is essential for long-term success in your weight-loss journey. Remember, setbacks are not failures—they are chances to learn, grow, and improve.

Strategies for Staying on Track After a Slip-Up.

Staying on track after a slip-up in your weight-loss journey involves a combination of self-compassion, strategic planning, and practical steps to regain momentum. Here are some effective strategies:

1. Acknowledge and Accept the Slip-Up

> Recognize the Incident: Understand that slip-ups are normal and part of the process. Acknowledge what happened without judgment.

> Accept Imperfection: Accept that perfection is unrealistic, and slip-ups do not define your entire journey.

2. Reflect and Learn

> Analyze the Trigger: Reflect on what caused the slip-up. Was it stress, emotional eating, lack of preparation, or social situations?

> Identify Patterns: Look for patterns in your behavior that might lead to slip-ups, and think about how you can address these triggers in the future.

3. Practice Self-Compassion

Be Kind to Yourself: Treat yourself with kindness and understanding. Avoid negative self-talk and remember that everyone makes mistakes.

Focus on Positives: Reflect on your overall progress and the positive changes you've made so far.

4. Recommit to Your Goals

Revisit Your Why: Remind yourself of the reasons why you embarked on your weight-loss journey. Reconnecting with your motivation can help you regain focus.

Set Fresh Goals: Establish new, achievable short-term goals to create momentum. These can be as simple as drinking more water, getting enough sleep, or planning meals for the week.

5. Plan and Prepare

Meal Planning: Plan your meals and snacks in advance to avoid impulsive eating. Stock up on healthy foods and keep tempting items out of the house.

Exercise Schedule: Create a realistic exercise plan that fits into your schedule. Include activities you enjoy to make it more sustainable.

6. Seek Support

Talk to Friends or Family: Share your experiences with trusted friends or family members who can offer support and encouragement.

Join a Support Group: Consider joining a weight-loss support group, either in person or online, to connect with others who understand your challenges.

7. Implement Small, Positive Changes

Gradual Adjustments: Start with small, manageable changes to ease back into your routine. For example, add an extra serving of vegetables to your meals or take a short walk each day.

Daily Goals: Set small, daily goals that are easy to achieve and can build confidence.

8. Use Tools and Resources

Track Progress: Use a journal, app, or spreadsheet to track your food intake, exercise, and progress. This can help you stay accountable and aware of your habits.

Educational Resources: Educate yourself about nutrition and healthy habits to make informed choices.

9. Stay Positive and Persistent

Positive Affirmations: Use positive affirmations to boost your confidence and remind yourself of your capabilities.

Persistent Effort: Understand that persistence is key. Consistently putting in effort, even after setbacks, is crucial for long-term success.

10. Celebrate Small Wins

Acknowledge Progress: Celebrate small victories along the way. Whether it's losing a pound, sticking to your exercise plan, or making a healthy food choice, acknowledging these wins can boost your motivation.

Reward Yourself: Treat yourself to non-food rewards, such as a new workout outfit, a massage, or a fun activity, to reinforce positive behavior.

Example Scenario: How to Get Back on Track

Situation: You attended a party and overindulged in high-calorie foods and drinks.

Step-by-Step Recovery Plan:

1. Acknowledge: Accept that you overindulged and understand that it's a normal part of the journey.

2. Reflect: Think about why you overindulged. Was it due to peer pressure, lack of healthy options, or emotional triggers?

3. Recommit: Reaffirm your commitment to your weight-loss goals. Remind yourself why you started and what you hope to achieve.

4. Plan: Prepare a healthy meal plan for the next few days to ensure you have nutritious options readily available. Include plenty of vegetables, lean proteins, and whole grains.

5. Exercise: Schedule some enjoyable physical activities, such as a walk in the park, a yoga class, or a bike ride, to help burn extra calories and improve your mood.

6. Support: Talk to a friend or family member about your experience. They can offer support and help keep you accountable.

7. Celebrate: If you make it through the next few days sticking to your plan, reward yourself with a non-food treat, like a new book or a movie night.

By using these strategies, you can effectively stay on track after a slip-up and continue making progress toward your weight-loss goals. Remember, setbacks are temporary, and each day is a new opportunity to make positive choices.

Chapter 5

Developing Healthy Habits

Creating a Sustainable Routine

The Power of Small, Consistent Changes: Small changes add up over time. Focus on making one small change at a time, and let these build into lasting habits.

Embarking on a weight-loss journey involves more than just diet and exercise; it requires breaking bad habits, identifying triggers and obstacles, and adopting healthier behaviors. Here are some strategies to help you along the way:

Breaking Bad Habits

1. Recognize and Understand Your Habits:

> Identify Bad Habits: List the habits that negatively impact your weight-loss goals, such as late-night snacking, overeating, or skipping workouts.

> Understand the Habit Loop: Each habit consists of a cue (trigger), routine (behavior), and reward. Understanding this loop can help you identify how to change it.

2. Replace Bad Habits with Healthy Ones:

Substitute with Positive Behaviors: Replace unhealthy habits with healthier alternatives. For example, replace late-night snacking with a relaxing bedtime routine like reading or meditating.

Gradual Changes: Make gradual changes to avoid feeling overwhelmed. Start with one habit at a time and build on your successes.

3. Set Specific Goals:

Clear and Achievable Goals: Set clear, specific, and achievable goals. For example, instead of "eat healthier," aim for "include a serving of vegetables in every meal."

Short-Term and Long-Term Goals: Break down your long-term weight loss goal into smaller, short-term goals to keep motivated and track progress.

Identifying Triggers and Obstacles

1. Identify Triggers:

Keep a Journal: Track your eating habits, emotions, and activities to identify patterns and triggers that lead to unhealthy behaviors.

Common Triggers: Recognize common triggers such as stress, boredom, social situations, or certain times of the day.

2. Identify Obstacles:

List Obstacles: List the obstacles that hinder your progress, such as lack of time, lack of motivation, or environmental factors.

Analyze Obstacles: Understand why these obstacles occur and how they affect your behavior.

Practical Tips for Overcoming Unhealthy Behaviors

1. Plan and Prepare:

Meal Planning: Plan your meals and snacks for the week. Prepare healthy meals in advance to avoid relying on unhealthy convenience foods.

Healthy Snacks: Keep healthy snacks like fruits, nuts, or yogurt on hand to avoid unhealthy choices.

2. Create a Supportive Environment:

Remove Temptations: Keep unhealthy foods out of the house and stock up on healthy options.

Support System: Surround yourself with supportive friends and family who encourage your healthy habits. Consider joining a support group.

3. Manage Stress and Emotions:

Stress Management Techniques: Practice stress management techniques like deep breathing, meditation, yoga, or physical activity.

Healthy Emotional Coping: Find healthy ways to cope with emotions, such as talking to a friend, journaling, or engaging in a hobby.

4. Establish a Routine:

Consistent Schedule: Establish a consistent eating and exercise schedule to create a routine.

Sleep Hygiene: Ensure you get enough sleep, as lack of sleep can lead to poor food choices and decreased motivation for exercise.

5. Stay Accountable:

Track Progress: Use a journal, app, or spreadsheet to track your food intake, exercise, and progress.

Regular Check-Ins: Regularly check in with a friend, family member, or coach to discuss your progress and challenges.

6. Reward Yourself:

Non-Food Rewards: Reward yourself with non-food items or activities when you reach your goals. This can help reinforce positive behavior.

7. Be Patient and Persistent:

Consistency Over Perfection: Focus on consistency rather than perfection. It's okay to have setbacks; what matters is getting back on track.

Celebrate Small Wins: Celebrate small achievements to stay motivated and remind yourself of your progress.

Example Scenario: Overcoming Late-Night Snacking

1. Identify the Habit:

> Habit: Late-night snacking.

> Cue: Feeling bored or stressed in the evening.

> Routine: Eating unhealthy snacks while watching TV.

> Reward: Temporary comfort or distraction.

2. Replace the Habit:

> New Routine: Develop a relaxing bedtime routine, such as reading a book, taking a warm bath, or practicing meditation.

> New Reward: Feeling relaxed and ready for sleep.

3. Plan and Prepare:

> Keep healthy snacks like sliced veggies or a small portion of nuts available if you need a snack.

> Avoid keeping high-calorie, high-sugar snacks in the house.

4. Create a Supportive Environment:

> Set a specific time to stop eating each evening, such as 8 PM.

> Inform family members of your new routine to gain their support.

5. Manage Stress and Emotions:

Practice stress-relief techniques during the day to reduce overall stress levels.

Engage in an evening activity that you find enjoyable and relaxing.

By implementing these strategies, you can break bad habits, overcome triggers and obstacles, and develop healthier behaviors that support your weight-loss journey. Remember that consistency, patience, and self-compassion are key components of long-term success.

Chapter 6

Navigating Social Situations

Eating Out and Social Events

Making healthier choices at restaurants.

Balancing enjoyment and discipline at parties.

Navigating restaurants and social events can be challenging when you're on a weight-loss journey. However, with a bit of planning and mindfulness, you can enjoy these occasions without derailing your progress. Here's how:

Making Healthier Choices at Restaurants

1. Plan Ahead:

> Research Menus: Look up the restaurant's menu online before you go and decide on a healthy option in advance.

> Eat Light Before: Have a light snack or meal before going out to avoid arriving excessively hungry.

2. Be Mindful of Portions:

Share Dishes: Split entrees or appetizers with a friend to control portion sizes.

Ask for Half Portions: Some restaurants will serve half portions if you ask.

Box Half: Ask for a to-go box at the beginning of the meal and pack away half of your meal immediately.

3. Choose Healthier Options:

Lean Proteins: Opt for grilled, baked, or steamed proteins like chicken, fish, or tofu instead of fried or breaded options.

Vegetables: Fill at least half of your plate with vegetables. Choose salads, steamed veggies, or stir-fries.

Whole Grains: Select whole grains such as brown rice, quinoa, or whole-wheat pasta over refined grains.

Dressings and Sauces: Request dressings and sauces on the side and use them sparingly. Opt for olive oil and vinegar over creamy dressings.

4. Drink Smart:

Water First: Start with a glass of water. It helps with satiety and hydration.

Limit Alcohol: Alcohol can add unnecessary calories. If you drink, choose lighter options like wine or spirits with low-calorie mixers, and set a limit.

5. Special Requests:

Customize Orders: Don't be afraid to ask for modifications, such as grilling instead of frying or substituting a side of fries with a salad.

Hold the Bread: Skip the breadbasket or limit yourself to one piece.

Balancing Enjoyment and Discipline at Parties

1. Mindful Eating:

Survey the Options: Take a look at all the available food before filling your plate. This helps you choose what you truly want to eat.

Portion Control: Use a smaller plate and take modest portions. You can always go back for more if you're still hungry.

Pace Yourself: Eat slowly and savor each bite. It takes time for your body to register fullness.

2. Choose Wisely:

Protein and Veggies First: Focus on protein-rich foods and vegetables before moving on to other options.

Healthy Options: Look for healthier choices such as grilled meats, vegetable platters, and salads.

Limit High-Calorie Foods: Enjoy treats in moderation. Take a small portion of high-calorie dishes like desserts or creamy dips.

3. Stay Hydrated:

Drink Water: Keep a glass of water in hand to stay hydrated and reduce the temptation to overeat.

Watch Alcohol Intake: If you choose to drink, alternate alcoholic beverages with water or club soda to pace yourself.

4. Stay Active:

Socialize Away from Food: Engage in conversations and activities away from the food table.

Get Moving: If the party has dancing or games, participate to stay active and burn some extra calories.

5. Bring a Healthy Dish:

Contribute a Healthy Option: If it's a potluck or gathering where you can bring a dish, prepare something healthy that you enjoy. This ensures there will be at least one nutritious option available.

Maintaining a Positive Mindset

1. Balance and Moderation: Remember that one meal or event won't derail your progress. Enjoy yourself in moderation and get back on track with your next meal.

2. Plan Ahead: If you know you'll be indulging, plan lighter meals and more exercise earlier in the day.

3. Focus on Social Aspects: Shift your focus from food to the social aspects of events. Enjoy the company, conversations, and activities.

4. Forgive Slip-Ups: If you overeat, don't dwell on it. Acknowledge it, learn from it, and move on without guilt.

By making conscious choices and balancing enjoyment with discipline, you can navigate eating out and social events while staying committed to your weight-loss goals.

Building a Support System
Finding supportive friends and communities.
The importance of accountability partners.

Finding Supportive Friends and Communities

1. Join Local Groups: Look for weight-loss support groups, fitness classes, or wellness workshops in your area. Community centers, gyms, and health clubs often host such events.

2. Online Communities: There are many online forums, social media groups, and websites dedicated to weight-loss support. Sites like Reddit, MyFitnessPal, and Facebook have active communities where members share tips, success stories, and encouragement.

3. Fitness Apps: Many fitness apps have built-in communities where users can interact, share progress, and motivate each other. Apps like Fitbit, Strava, and Noom offer such features.

4. Friends and Family: Talk to your friends and family about your goals. They can offer support, join you with others in your activities, and help keep you accountable.

5. Professional Support: Consider joining a program led by a nutritionist, dietitian, or personal trainer. They can provide expert advice and connect you with others on similar journeys.

The Importance of Accountability Partners

1. Motivation: An accountability partner can provide the extra push you need to stay motivated, especially on days when you feel like giving up.

2. Consistency: Having someone to check in with regularly can help you stay consistent with your diet and exercise routines.

3. Shared Goals: Working towards common goals with a partner can make the process more enjoyable and less daunting. You can celebrate each other's successes and support each other through challenges.

4. Perspective and Advice: Accountability partners can offer new perspectives, advice, and constructive feedback. They can help you see things you might have missed and suggest new strategies.

5. Emotional Support: Weight-loss journeys can be emotionally challenging. An accountability partner can provide emotional support, helping you stay positive and focused.

Tips for Building a Support System

1. Be Open: Share your goals, struggles, and progress with your support network. Openness encourages others to offer their help and support.

2. Set Clear Expectations: Communicate your needs and expectations clearly with your accountability partner(s). This helps avoid misunderstandings and ensures that everyone is on the same page.

3. Regular Check-ins: Schedule regular check-ins with your accountability partner or support group. This could be daily, weekly, or monthly, depending on what works best for you.

4. Be Supportive in Return: Support is a two-way street. Offer encouragement and help to others in your support network. This builds stronger, reciprocal relationships.

5. Celebrate Milestones: Celebrate your achievements, no matter how small. Recognizing progress can boost morale and keep everyone motivated.

Building a support system can make a significant difference in achieving your weight-loss goals. With the right people at your side, you'll find the journey more manageable and rewarding.

Chapter 8

Celebrating Milestones

Recognizing Achievements

The importance of celebrating small victories.
Non-food rewards to motivate yourself.
Reflecting on your journey
Writing a letter to your past self.
Visualizing your future self and continued success.

Letter to My Past Self

Dear Past Self,

I hope this letter finds you well. You are about to embark on an incredible journey of transformation and self-discovery. I know you have your doubts and fears, but let me assure you, everything you're about to experience will be worth it.

When you first decided to lose weight, it wasn't just about the numbers on the scale; it was about reclaiming your health, confidence, and happiness. The beginning will be challenging. You'll face temptations, setbacks, and moments of self-doubt. But each of these obstacles will only make you stronger and more resilient.

Remember the first time you went for a run and felt like giving up after just a few minutes? Or when you chose a salad over your usual comfort food and questioned if it was all worth it? Those small decisions, repeated consistently, will lead to significant changes. You'll learn that progress isn't always linear, but each step, no matter how small, is a step forward.

Celebrate the victories, both big and small. The first time you notice your clothes fitting better, the moment you realize you have more energy, and the compliments from friends and family who notice your transformation – these are all milestones to cherish. Don't forget to appreciate the non-scale victories as well, like improved sleep, reduced stress, and newfound confidence.

Stay patient and be kind to yourself. There will be days when you slip up, and that's okay. What matters is how you pick yourself up and keep moving forward. Surround yourself with supportive people who uplift you and share in your successes and struggles.

Most importantly, remember why you started. Keep that vision of your healthier, happier self in mind, and let it guide you through the tough times. You're capable of so much more than you think, and I'm proud of the person you're becoming.

With determination and love,

Your Future Self

Visualization of Future Self

Close your eyes and picture yourself a year from now. Imagine waking up in the morning with a sense of accomplishment and pride. You look in the mirror and see a reflection of someone who has worked hard, stayed committed, and achieved remarkable progress.

Your days are filled with energy and enthusiasm. You move with confidence, knowing that your body is stronger and healthier. The activities that once seemed daunting are now a regular part of your routine. You enjoy a balanced diet, savoring the flavors of wholesome foods that nourish your body and soul.

Visualize yourself setting new fitness goals and achieving them. Whether it's running a 5k, lifting heavier weights, or mastering a new yoga pose, you embrace the challenges with determination and excitement. You've built a sustainable lifestyle that allows you to enjoy life to the fullest, without the constraints of past habits.

See yourself inspiring others with your journey. Friends, family, and even strangers look to you as a source of motivation. Your story becomes a testament to what's possible with dedication and perseverance.

Feel the sense of inner peace and self-acceptance. You've learned to love yourself at every stage of your journey, understanding that true health and happiness come from within. Your journey has not only transformed your body but also your mind and spirit.

As you continue to grow, you set new goals, knowing that the sky's the limit. You embrace the future with optimism and excitement, confident in your ability to overcome any obstacles and achieve lasting success.

Embrace this vision and let it guide you forward. Your future self is waiting, proud and ready to celebrate every victory along the way.

Chapter 9

Maintenance and Beyond

Transitioning to Maintenance Mode

Adjusting your diet and exercise for long-term success.

Transitioning to maintenance in the context of diet and exercise means shifting your focus from losing weight or building muscle to maintaining your current weight and fitness levels. This involves making adjustments to your diet and exercise routines to create a sustainable, long-term lifestyle. Here's what it generally entails:

1. Diet Adjustments:

Caloric Intake: Adjust your caloric intake to match your maintenance level, where calories consumed equal calories burned.

Balanced Nutrition: Ensure your diet includes a balance of macronutrients (proteins, fats, carbohydrates) and micronutrients (vitamins, minerals) to support overall health.

Portion Control: Continue practicing portion control to avoid overeating.

Flexibility: Allow for occasional indulgences to make the diet sustainable in the long term.

2. Exercise Adjustments:

Consistency: Maintain a consistent exercise routine to keep your fitness levels stable.

Variety: Incorporate a variety of activities to prevent boredom and reduce the risk of injury.

Intensity: Adjust the intensity of workouts to a level that is challenging but not exhausting, ensuring sustainability.

Rest and Recovery: Prioritize rest and recovery to prevent burnout and injuries.

3. Lifestyle Integration:

Habits: Develop healthy habits that can be maintained without significant effort, such as regular meal planning and physical activity.

Mindset: Shift your mindset from short-term goals to long-term health and well-being.

Monitoring: Regularly monitor your weight, body composition, and overall health to make small adjustments as needed.

4. Flexibility and Adaptation:

Adjustments: Be prepared to adjust your diet and exercise routines as your body and lifestyle change over time.

Realistic Goals: Set realistic, achievable goals that focus on maintaining health rather than perfection.

By transitioning to maintenance with these adjustments, you can create a balanced and sustainable approach to diet and exercise that supports long-term success.

Staying Vigilant About Old Habits.

Staying vigilant about old habits on your weight-loss journey is essential to ensuring long-term success. Here are some strategies to help you stay aware of and manage old habits:

1. Awareness and Monitoring

Track Your Habits

Journaling: Keep a daily journal of your eating habits, physical activity, and emotional state. This will help you identify patterns and triggers that lead to old habits resurfacing.

Apps and Tools: Use apps to track your food intake, exercise, and progress. Many apps offer reminders and insights that can keep you on track.

Regular Self-Check-Ins

Weekly Reviews: Set aside time each week to review your progress, successes, and areas where old habits might be creeping back in.

Monthly Goals: Reassess your goals and adjust them as needed to stay focused and motivated.

2. Identify Triggers

Understand Your Triggers

Emotional Triggers: Recognize emotions that lead to old habits, such as stress, boredom, or sadness. Knowing your emotional triggers helps you prepare and develop healthier coping mechanisms.

Environmental Triggers: Identify situations or environments that prompt old habits, such as social events, specific locations, or times of day.

Plan for Triggers

Coping Strategies: Develop strategies to cope with triggers. For example, if stress leads to overeating, try stress-reduction techniques like meditation, deep breathing, or going for a walk.

Avoid Temptations: Make changes to your environment to reduce temptations. Keep healthy snacks readily available and remove unhealthy options from your home.

3. Replace Old Habits with New Ones

Healthy Substitutions

Swap Foods: Replace unhealthy foods with nutritious alternatives. For example, swap chips for veggie sticks or fruit.

Positive Activities: Replace sedentary activities with physical ones. Instead of watching TV when bored, go for a walk, do a quick workout, or engage in a hobby.

Consistency is Key

Routine: Establish a consistent daily routine that includes healthy eating, regular physical activity, and self-care practices.

Gradual Changes: Make small, incremental changes rather than drastic overhauls. This makes new habits more sustainable and less overwhelming.

4. Stay Motivated

Revisit Your Goals and Motivations

Visual Reminders: Keep visual reminders of your goals, such as a vision board, motivational quotes, or progress photos.

Reflect on Your Why: Regularly remind yourself of why you started your weight-loss journey. Reflecting on your motivations can reignite your commitment.

Celebrate Successes

Small Wins: Celebrate small milestones along the way. Recognize and reward your

Continuing to Grow

Setting new health and fitness goals.

Continuing to grow and setting new health and fitness goals is essential for sustaining motivation and progress on a weight-loss journey. Here are some strategies and tips to help you stay on track and keep advancing:

1. Review and Reflect

> Evaluate Your Progress: Regularly assess your progress by tracking metrics such as weight, body measurements, fitness levels, and how your clothes fit.

> Celebrate Achievements: Recognize and celebrate the milestones you have reached, no matter how small they might seem.

2. Set Specific and Realistic Goals

> SMART Goals: Ensure your goals are Specific, Measurable, Achievable, Relevant, and Time-bound. For example, "I will lose 5 pounds in the next month by exercising five times a week and following a balanced diet."

> Short-term and Long-term Goals: Set both short-term (weekly/monthly) and long-term (6 months/year) goals to keep you motivated and focused.

3. Diversify Your Workouts

> Try New Activities: Incorporate a variety of exercises to keep things interesting. This could include strength training, cardio, yoga, Pilates, or dance classes.

Progressive Overload: Gradually increase the intensity, duration, or complexity of your workouts to continue challenging your body.

4. Nutrition Goals

Balanced Diet: Aim for a balanced diet rich in whole foods, including fruits, vegetables, lean proteins, healthy fats, and whole grains.

Hydration: Make sure you stay well-hydrated by drinking plenty of water throughout the day.

Mindful Eating: Practice mindful eating to better understand your hunger and fullness cues, and to make more intentional food choices.

5. Behavioral and Lifestyle Goals

Sleep: Aim for 7-9 hours of quality sleep each night as it plays a crucial role in weight management and overall health.

Stress Management: Incorporate stress-reducing activities such as meditation, deep breathing exercises, or hobbies you enjoy.

Consistency: Focus on building sustainable habits rather than seeking quick fixes. Consistency is key for long-term success.

6. Track and Adjust

Use Tools: Utilize apps, journals, or trackers to monitor your food intake, exercise, and progress.

Be Flexible: If a particular approach isn't working, be open to trying new methods or adjusting your goals.

7. Seek Support

Join a Community: Engage with online or local fitness communities for support, motivation, and accountability.

Professional Guidance: Consider working with a personal trainer, nutritionist, or health coach for personalized advice and encouragement.

8. Mental and Emotional Health

Positive Mindset: Maintain a positive attitude towards your journey. Focus on what your body can do rather than just the numbers on the scale.

Self-Compassion: Be kind to yourself and recognize that setbacks are a natural part of the process. Use them as learning opportunities rather than reasons to give up.

By incorporating these strategies, you can continue to grow, set new health and fitness goals, and make sustained progress on your weight-loss journey.

Exploring new Hobbies and Activities to Stay Engaged

Embarking on a weight-loss journey can be challenging, but incorporating new hobbies and activities can make it more enjoyable and engaging. Here are some ideas to keep you motivated and entertained:

Physical Activities

1. Hiking: Enjoy the outdoors and burn calories by exploring local trails.

2. Dancing: Join a dance class or follow online tutorials. It's a fun way to exercise.

3. Yoga or Pilates: These activities help with flexibility, strength, and relaxation.

4. Cycling: Ride a bike around your neighborhood or explore bike trails.

5. Swimming: A low-impact exercise that works out the entire body.

6. Team Sports: Join a local league for soccer, basketball, or volleyball.

Creative Hobbies

1. Cooking and Healthy Baking: Experiment with new recipes and learn to make nutritious meals.

2. Photography: Capture your weight-loss journey and the beautiful places you explore.

3. Gardening: Grow your own fruits and vegetables, which can also support healthy eating.

4. Painting or Drawing: Express yourself creatively and de-stress.

5. Writing or Journaling: Document your progress and reflect on your journey.

Educational Activities

1. Reading: Dive into books on nutrition, fitness, or any topic that interests you.

2. Learning a New Language: Use apps or take classes to learn a new language.

3. Online Courses: Enroll in courses that interest you, from cooking to coding.

Social Activities

1. Join a Club: Find local clubs or online groups that share your interests.

2. Volunteer: Offer your time to causes you care about and stay active.

3. Attend Workshops: Look for workshops on fitness, nutrition, or personal development.

Mindfulness and Relaxation

1. Mindfulness: Practice mindfulness to enhance your ability to stay present and reduce stress. Mindfulness involves being fully engaged with the current moment, whether it's through paying close attention to the sensation of water while washing dishes or the sounds you hear during a walk. It ranges from simple attentiveness to more deliberate practices.

2. Meditation: Explore various forms of meditation to achieve relaxation and focus. Meditation encompasses different techniques, including guided relaxation, transcendental meditation, mantra chanting, Yoga Nidra (a form of meditation without movement), and Non-Sleep Deep Rest Meditation. Each method offers unique benefits, contributing to relaxation and overall well-being.

3. Reading Self-Help Books: Gain new insights and strategies for personal growth through self-help literature.

4. Listening to Podcasts: Find inspiring and educational podcasts related to health and wellness to support your journey.

Combining Interests

1. Travel: Plan active vacations that include hiking, biking, or exploring new places.

2. Fitness Challenges: Join or create fitness challenges with friends or online communities.

3. Creating a Blog or Vlog: Share your weight-loss journey and hobbies with others.

Staying engaged with these activities can help you remain motivated, reduce stress, and make your weight-loss journey more enjoyable.

Conclusion

Every weight-loss journey is unique and filled with its own challenges and triumphs. Remember, the goal is not just to lose weight but to gain a healthier, happier you. Keep pushing forward, stay patient with yourself, and celebrate every step of your progress. This journey is about becoming the best version of yourself, and you're already on your way.

As I look back on this incredible journey to a healthier me, I am filled with a sense of accomplishment and gratitude. What started as a challenging endeavor has transformed into a lifestyle that brings me joy, vitality, and confidence. This journey was not just about losing weight but about gaining a deeper understanding of myself, my body, and the importance of perseverance.

Throughout this process, I have learned that true health extends beyond physical appearance. It encompasses mental well-being, emotional resilience, and a positive outlook on life. The support of my family, friends, and community has been invaluable, reminding me that we are never alone in our struggles or triumphs.

The road to a healthier me was paved with setbacks and victories, moments of doubt, and bursts of inspiration. Each step, no matter how small, contributed to the larger picture of my transformation. Embracing healthier habits, making mindful choices, and prioritizing self-care have become integral parts of my daily routine.

To anyone embarking on their own journey to better health, I offer this advice: be patient with yourself, celebrate your progress, and never underestimate the power of determination. Change is a gradual process, and every effort counts. Remember that setbacks are not failures but opportunities to learn and grow stronger.

As this chapter of my story comes to an end, I am excited about the future and the continued evolution of my health journey. The lessons I have learned and the habits I have cultivated will stay with me, guiding me towards a life of sustained wellness and happiness.

Thank you for joining me on this journey. Here's to a healthier, happier future for us all

This book is meant to be a companion, offering practical advice and heartfelt encouragement as you navigate your own path to better health. Your journey is worth it, and so are you.